FOR MY FAVORITE

sex partner

LET'S MAKE LOVE
THEN HAVE HOT DIRTY SEX

①

Masturbate in front of me

additional details :

Talk about your experience :

LET'S MAKE LOVE
THEN HAVE HOT DIRTY SEX

②

Bend over a chair
and invite me
to take you

additional details :

....

....

....

....

Talk about your experience :

LET'S MAKE LOVE
THEN HAVE HOT DIRTY SEX

③

additional details :

....

....

....

....

Talk about your experience :

LET'S MAKE LOVE
THEN HAVE HOT DIRTY SEX

(4)

additional details :

....

....

....

....

Talk about your experience :

LET'S MAKE LOVE
THEN HAVE HOT DIRTY SEX

5

Get naked in the pool and
give me a blowjob underwater
or give me
a hand job while I enjoy the view

additional details :

Talk about your experience :

LET'S MAKE LOVE
THEN HAVE HOT DIRTY SEX

6

Surprise me with
quickie sex at work

additional details :

Talk about your experience :

LET'S MAKE LOVE
THEN HAVE HOT DIRTY SEX

7

additional details :

....

....

....

....

Talk about your experience :

LET'S MAKE LOVE
THEN HAVE HOT DIRTY SEX

8

additional details :

Talk about your experience :

LET'S MAKE LOVE
THEN HAVE HOT DIRTY SEX

⑨

what is your deepest,
darkest fantasy... I'm gonna
make it come true!

additional details :

....

....

....

....

Talk about your experience :

LET'S MAKE LOVE
THEN HAVE HOT DIRTY SEX

10

Making love discreetly
at a party

additional details :
....
....
....
....

Talk about your experience :

additional details :

....

....

....

....

Talk about your experience :

LET'S MAKE LOVE
THEN HAVE HOT DIRTY SEX

12

additional details :

....

....

....

....

Talk about your experience :

LET'S MAKE LOVE
THEN HAVE HOT DIRTY SEX

13

jerk me off with your tits and look me in the eye.

additional details :

....

....

....

Talk about your experience :

LET'S MAKE LOVE
THEN HAVE HOT DIRTY SEX

14

tomorrow you'll wake me up with a blowjob.

additional details :

Talk about your experience :

LET'S MAKE LOVE
THEN HAVE HOT DIRTY SEX

15

additional details :

Talk about your experience :

LET'S MAKE LOVE
THEN HAVE HOT DIRTY SEX

16

additional details :

Talk about your experience :

LET'S MAKE LOVE
THEN HAVE HOT DIRTY SEX

17

watch a porn
movie together

additional details :

....
....
....
....

Talk about your experience :

LET'S MAKE LOVE
THEN HAVE HOT DIRTY SEX

18

tomorrow you'll
wake me up with a
blowjob.

additional details :

Talk about your experience :

LET'S MAKE LOVE
THEN HAVE HOT DIRTY SEX

19

Doing a sexy photo shoot together

additional details :

....

....

....

....

Talk about your experience :

LET'S MAKE LOVE
THEN HAVE HOT DIRTY SEX

20

additional details :

Talk about your experience :

9 781659 800814